A Stargazer Publication

ISBN - 9781095403570
Please go to http://www.thecombinationofthings.com
to sign up for our newsletter announcing new releases.

Editor - Cynthia Calzone

Cover photo - Laura Pedrick

Cover Design - Noel Sellon

THE COMBINATION OF THINGS

By

Gary S. Patterson

THE COMBINATION OF THINGS

It's been a lock that's taken me a long time to unlock
and open up to see the secret within.

That's life. I think that's true of most people.
The journey is an algorithm, a puzzle to be solved.
A recipe for the right number of ingredients, the right combin-
ation to unlock the desired flavor.
Stir gently.
Repeat daily.
Patience is the key.
Exercise will induce calmness and pay attention to improving
HRV.
Reap results slowly over time.

Now I take the stairs two at a time and sing for no reason! Stay
with me, and you can do the same!
And yes, I do all the stuff in this book!

TABLE OF CONTENTS

INTRODUCTION

This is my first book. I'd always thought I was going to write the great American novel when I was in school, but life got in the way as it often does for most people.
I was no different.

I ran track and cross-country in high school and played Little League baseball all the way through to the majors. Football in the backyard ... I was a star, never bothered going out for the high school team though. Back then we didn't dream of playing in the NFL. At least I didn't. I was way too busy. When I got home from school, I had a paper route to attend to, cycling three to four miles a day to deliver all my papers.

I was also in the Cub Scouts and Boy Scouts, which took up increasingly more time on the weekends as I became a patrol leader and eventually earned Eagle Scout status. I also studied with my Minister for 2 years and achieved the God and Country award. This is an award only several hundred Boy Scouts nation-wide have ever earned, so it took quite a bit of effort on my part and culminated with me giving several speeches in front of a full church congregation and public talks for parents and friends.

All the while I was affected by asthma from early on, at times it would leave me alone and then like a phantom, visit me in the night and attack. It was a mysterious thing, and doctors had no suggestions back in the 60s except that perhaps we should move to Arizona.

I went off to college and became immersed in the 1960's hip-pie lifestyle; drinking, smoking cigarettes, marijuana and taking various alternative substances. A friend got carted off in an am-bulance dead from a heroin overdose, so right off the bat, I decided that wasn't for me.

The next couple of years saw me get kicked out of several colleges for various reasons. Bad grades, drugs, you name it.

I was searching for a purpose to life and having a hard time finding it. It seemed to be so easy for other people.
If you're reading this, it wasn't probably easy for you either.

I often felt like I was on an island. And really unable to describe my situation.

If you ever felt this way, the pages that follow may sound familiar to you, but I think some of the methods I've discovered are new and unique. Not that I invented them myself, but my goal here is to give them a wider mainstream exposure.

Because if you don't have your health, what do you have?

Pain, anxiety, and maybe turbulence in your business personal and professional life? Suffer in silence?
Probably.

Anyway, unless you're a super bio-hacker, if you read on, I guarantee you will find something within these pages that you never knew before.

WHO IS THIS BOOK FOR?

You may have a chronic condition like me which has been treated with limited success by your traditional medical caregiver. Maybe no success. Maybe you are just on a maintenance regimen.

You want to lose weight but can't stick to a diet.

It's my belief that if you don't have a chronic disease or illness or affliction that you're dealing with already, the way things are today with the state of our food supply and environment, you'll soon acquire one. So, in that sense, this book is for everyone.

BACK PAIN 101

This book is for those of you who have reached the end of your rope with traditional "cures" for your constant back pain. I'm going to tell you right up front you should consider and consult your current family doctor or medical professional before trying or embracing any of the fixes put forward in this book. That being said, I'm sure if you've reached the point where you're reading this book, you're ready to try just about anything.

I see commercials and advertisements in print publications and on television every day advertising the latest gizmo or gadget or potion lotion or the latest treatment for lower or mid-back pain. Now at this point in my life, I know that these are just stopgap measures and are not really addressing the root of the problem. What I have set forth here are several approaches, both exercise-wise, static-wise, and nutritionally that have worked for me. These by no means may work for everyone and notice I use the word fix and not cure because most of these methods that I present in this book are those that will have to be practiced either daily or several times a week to continue the desired effects. Everyone is different, and every case is different. That is why I include nutritional information along with these exercises and procedures because, without the proper nourishment, our bodies cannot hope to repair themselves to their maximum ability. Also, I have included illustrations for many of the exercises and postures to help get you on your way. These are by no means an endpoint, but simply a place to start. The idea is to keep it basic and simple so that you can maintain a routine that is quick and concise, and hopefully able to be shoe-horned into your busy day. I find that exercise is better done in the morning or early day on an empty stomach so that your body is not distracted by the digestion of food. More on that in its own chapter.

To wrap up this intro, I just want to say that the information contained in this book has been gained from many years of experimentation on my part. You'll not find any peer-reviewed studies presented here. The solutions offered in this book are not monetarily worth the time of the companies who would normally fund these types of studies. Hence, no money to be made, no studies. The bottom line is if you're reading this book you've probably had all the so-called professional medical advice you can stand and you're ready to take matters into your own hands. And believe me, you can! I am living proof of that!

WHY AM I QUALIFIED TO
WRITE THIS BOOK?

1. At five-years-old, in the middle of the night while on a weekend visit to my Dad's Aunt's farm in Milford, Delaware, I had my first episode of non-breathing. My parents whisked me to the nearest emergency room where they shot me up with adrenaline, and it was announced that I had asthma. My better memories of that weekend were of cows, hay, and the wooden churn that nearly wore me out making ice cream in the barn.

2. My childhood and teenage years were a roller-coaster of normalcy and midnight attacks by the asthma monster, panicky calls by my mother to the family doctor to alert him we were on our way and his sleepy calm demeanor as he inserted the huge cannister-size needle into my arm. The adrenaline washed over me like one of the turbulent seashore waves at Stone Harbor on an August afternoon. And so, it went most often that way. I ran on the track and cross-country teams and sang in the school chorus and church choir. No problems. Sometimes there was talk of us relocating to Arizona, but that wasn't really a serious consideration. I didn't realize it at the time, but the exercise was minimizing the severity of my asthma and keeping at bay the frequency of the attacks.

3. Check in with me during college and post-college time, and I was unbelievably smoking cigarettes and weed, which all seemed to oddly agree with me. Poof! No breathing problems here!

4. By my mid-twenties that all caught up with me and it was off to the doctors again.

5.   Then, of course, when I broke my back in a motorcycle accident that started me off on a whole new path.

BACK STORY

In today's world, a troublesome back can disrupt your daily routine in an untold number of ways.

In this book I will explain how to solve those problems you're experiencing, the sciatica muscle spasms, herniated discs, general arthritis and in general, lower back problems.

I will tell you the step-by-step story of how I came upon the ultimate solution for fixing my back.

After too many times of being asked by interested parties why I haven't written a book about this, I'm finally getting around to it. I guess sometimes you feel as though you're not really adding much to the program and it's really nothing new, but then again, I guess any new perspective on a subject that a relatively small percentage of the population has any knowledge of is a step forward.

Thirty years ago, I remember it was a sunny spring day. I had been rototilling gardens to earn part-time money for quite some time. I went out to a house in West Chester, Pennsylvania situated on about 2 acres of ground. After being instructed as to the size of the garden, I proceeded to prepare the ground with my rototiller, and when I was done I went inside, and the guy who would hire me offered me a beer which I gladly accepted since it was a hot afternoon. After two or three more beers, the conversation turned to motorcycles, of which I had a few, and he also had a new motorcycle in the garage. He said he was more than willing to let me try riding his brand-new OSA competition motocross bike and we fired it up. I took it out into the field behind his house and before I knew what it, I was doing 65 miles an hour and waist high in weeds. I soon came upon a huge ravine and went flying through the air and almost made it over to the other side, but I hit the embankment as my feet came off the pegs and my body took the impact straight up my back, and the bike flipped over the edge. At least I landed on the flat surface of the top edge, unconscious, then seeing stars for the first time in my life.

After his wife's order to help me to my feet, I went back to my car and drove off, ignoring her request for me to call an ambulance. I went home and laid in bed for several days before I realized it the pain was so severe that I had to go to the emergency room. By sheer coincidence my family doctor was on the shift and took x-rays, showing them to me while saying: "You're out of your mind! Take a look at this; I don't even have words to describe it." I looked at the x-ray and saw pieces of my vertebrae floating around in spinal fluid, and my three bottom disks squashed, looking like many dumbbells.

He said, "If you had come in immediately I could have put you in a back brace, but now it was too late." I asked him what could be done and he said to just go home and take some ibuprofen and get some rest. Wow, those were the good old days, no chance to get hooked on opiates. So, I went home and stayed in bed for a day or so. After that, I couldn't stand it anymore and decided to go back to work. We had a landscaping company back then; it was just a lot of physical backbreaking work that wouldn't wait. I suffered a permanent blowout of some oblique muscles on my right side of my back by lifting something which I had been told not to do.

Now it's not as though I never had a drink before, but this was really the beginning of my drinking career. Whiskey became my best friend, and I needed relief 24 hours a day, so whiskey, along with Advil became a regular regimen. This book is also the story of my journey of curbing and eventually eliminating my alcohol intake through natural means. Of course, all that was caused by my messed-up back. I had no one to blame but myself. But that was about to change.

The funny thing was, like many chiropractors and doctors I

visited, they all told me not to do any hard,
physical exercise. After attempting the hard, physical exercise anyway, I realized my back problems were not going to go away by themselves, and I experienced a half light bulb moment.

Over the years, yoga helped a lot and then in the mid-2000s I was searching the Internet and happened upon Inversion. Curious, I began to research more, and it became obvious to me that there was something to this.

I decided that I thought this was something that I've yet to explore. I had to try it! You know what they say about some testimonials on the Internet, they're funny, and they can't be believed. There were just too many stories, and they were too complex and detailed as people related their stories on how they had cured themselves.

I had the secret but didn't really know what to do with it; it'd been a long time coming, and I hadn't recognized that the answer was right under my nose. Only after I took the plunge and got the equipment did I realize that this would be a momentous occasion. It still took me months to set everything up and attempt the beginning of what would become a lifesaver for me. A lifetime for a lifetime practice.

Progress was slow at the beginning, but I've become accustomed to that pace after years of doing yoga exercises and saying that the games are slow yet progressive. Anyone who has done yoga knows that the exercises are initially painful to the point of seeming to be impossible.

MY FATHER'S MOTHER

As I sit here today writing this book and reflect back on those who have influenced me the most in my childhood, I would have to say it was my father's mother. She had a unique, overall perspective on the world. She wasn't an overly religious person nor was she non-religious. Her first husband left her after my father was born, so she was forced to recreate herself. She became a hat maker, and I remember as a young boy even after she had remarried, I would go to her hat shop on Friday afternoons before I stayed for the weekend and watch in wonder as she created hats for women on the 'fly,' right on their heads. She was always busy and to my amazement, in great demand.

Also, perhaps they came for the stories. For me, they made me dizzy, but maybe it was all the smoke in the shop. The stories that meandered like a backcountry
rivulet that always enticed with the thought that they might actually open into some meaningful conclusion of a visible river. When asked about an incident or particular person's situation, her eventual assessment was, "Well ... it was a combination of things!"

There were Atlantic crossings, jewels acquired thru luck or chicanery, crazy partying, a lot of breathless cigarette smoking, Conga lines at the clubs in Havana (where she loved to hang out) and the comings and goings of the acquainted and the unacquainted.

Neighbors, relatives past and present, and nicotine-fueled figments of her imagination. On TV in those days, the Burns and Allen show was one of my favorites. And I had the cigar smoking Pop-Pop Charlie and Cigarette Choo-choo with Helen the Hatmaker providing a comic counterpoint to Charlie's wry assessments of life. To me, she was just Nana.

Charlie would say, "Oh man, can that woman cook!" (she didn't) and Nana would respond, "So you don't like my cookin' eh?" and shake her fist in a mock wind-up whilst he was asking, "What particular cooking (pointing to his head) are you referring to?" and on and on they'd go.

One of my final and lasting memories of Nana was the time we baked a chocolate cake caused we were bored, and the Phillies game wasn't on yet. She was a BIG Phillies fan and knew all the players. In the mid to late '50s, with the exception of Richie Ashburn, it was like watching the follies, and she had grand fun with it. Anyway, she baked 2 layers, and we debated the type of icing. She decided to get creative, and somehow the icing wasn't thick enough or was it that the oven was tilted and the layers weren't symmetrical. Replete with icing, we gazed on our cake as the top layer proceeded to slide off the bottom layer. As she motioned for the cake to behave, her hand grazed the hanging layer, and she ended up with a handful of cake, which she immediately threw in my face. A full-on food fight ensued in which we demolished the kitchen, and in the process, ingested a few handfuls of cake. I playfully asked her how she had made such a fantastic cake.

As if on cue, she immediately launched into a rousing rendition of *She's coming around the mountain!* She loved to sing. At the conclusion of our fun, she said, "Dear boy, it's a combination of things!"

THE ENVIRONMENT

CELL SENESCENCE

Cellular senescence is a phenomenon by which normal cells cease to divide.

At the end of the day, your everyday life is about cell death. You may think you're beating the odds, having the time of your life with a SAD (standard American diet), but by the time you have passed the 25-30-year-old mark, the free pass is over as far as hormone peak output and youthful metabolic momentum. This approach and thinking, unfortunately, have you slotted in the *Has Been* file.

I cannot stress enough that we are being assaulted with environmental garbage at unprecedented levels. The list is almost too long to contemplate. Dirty water, dirty air, dirty soil and on and on. And by dirty, I mean polluted by materials of unknown decomposition, chemicals in our water and soil transferred to our food in unfathomable ways. The genetic modification of our food supply continues unabated as the general public is too distracted by everyday concerns like juggling payments for bills to stay above water.

What foods we ingest, even with good intentions, are secretly being manipulated on a genetic level like never before. So, it is imperative to protect ourselves and put up a line of defense as it were.

Inflammatory Networks during Cellular Senescence: Causes and ...

https://www.ncbi.nlm.nih.gov/pmc/articles/PMC2879478/

As noted in the above paper, chronic inflammation is the cause of most of the high profile 'diseases' of our time.

"Chronic inflammation, by contrast, is the continued presence (sometimes over many years) of pro-inflammatory factors at levels higher than baseline, but many fold lower than those found in acute inflammation. Chronically inflamed tissues are characterized by the presence of infiltrating lymphocytes and macrophages, abundant blood vessels, fibrosis, and often, tissue necrosis [1, 2]. Chronic inflammation, as measured by the serum levels of pro-inflammatory mediators near sites of pathology, is associated with many age-related pathophysiologic processes and diseases, including Alzheimer's disease, diabetes, atherosclerosis, osteoarthritis, and cancer, among others [3, 4] (Figure 1). Chronic inflammation is also associated with normal aging. For example, on average, there is a 2–4 fold increase in serum levels of pro-inflammatory mediators (e.g., interleukin (IL)-6 and tumor necrosis factor (TNF)α) in aged individuals (>50 years of age), compared to younger individuals [5, 6]. Moreover, individuals who experience unusually healthy aging – for example, healthy centenarians – typically have a lower inflammatory profile than frail centenarians [7] (or individuals that display obvious signs of aging and age-related disease). The inflammatory status of a tissue or plasma profile is determined by a balance between pro- and anti-inflammatory factors. For example, although both frail and healthy centenarians often have plasma levels of pro-inflammatory mediators that are higher than young individuals, healthy centenarians often also have increased levels of anti-inflammatory mediators (for example, cortisol and IL-10) and, overall, reduced chronic inflammation [7].

CELLULAR ASSAULT

Every moment of every day, your body is under assault from impurities and toxins in your environment that constantly cause damage on an intracellular scale. This is commonly referred to in the scientific community as 'reactive oxidative stress' (ROS). A small amount of this ROS is beneficial and stimulates your immune system. However, the level and amount of ROS that our cells are bombarded with are so overwhelming that it results in a type of cell damage that leads to innumerable life-threatening conditions. This is not even taking into account the copious amounts of nutritionally deficient 'foods' we punish our bodies with on a daily basis that compound the crisis. Yes, it is a crisis. And one that desperately needs the attention of every living being on our planet.

It is with this thought in mind that I want to emphasize the need for you to forget about thinking in terms of the RDA and thinking about cycling maximum nutrients sourced as organically as possible, fresh produce, and best quality natural supplements.

Cycling is important. Cells have a rhythm and pounding them continually with a flood of stimulating nutrients can cause them to lose effectiveness. So one or two days of deprivation is actually the setup to make your cells hungry and extremely receptive to maximally absorb and convert the next wave of nutrition.

THE DIET IN A NUTSHELL

This isn't a self-help book, but yet it is how health has been an obsession of mine from an early age. It's just been a progression of things added to my daily routine that has finally gotten me to the point where I can feel as though I'm reaching a successful physical plateau.
A healthy body can, therefore, become a healthy mind, but that also takes a lot of intelligent input.

At the onset, let me be clear about a few pre-conditions so that the information in this book can be beneficial to you. The following food items and living practices are excised from your daily routine. After a few months, occasional cheating is OK! We're not perfect here or aspiring to monkhood. But at the onset, you should follow these guidelines strictly:

NO SUGAR including all artificial sweeteners.
NO DAIRY except occasional organic eggs and organic imported hard cheese* - domestic is loaded with undisclosed ingredients
NO PROCESSED FOODS - IN GENERAL ANYTHING IN A BAG OR BOX (transfats) *also JUICES
NO MEAT except unprepared chicken or fish
NO VEGETABLE OILS except olive and coconut oil, almond, etc.

If you must have fruit, keep it to one serving per day. Apples are best, low glycemic. Blueberries are good too. Fruit, in general, is a better choice than your free market protein bars and other supposed 'good-for-you' snacks. Just limit the amount.

I have to say most of my diet falls into what is commonly referred to these days as Paleo or Ketogenic. Try to eat whole foods.

PALEO OR KETO?

To start with, let's keep in mind that the Paleo Diet is based on a hunter grazer theory dating back to the beginning of mankind. As such it prohibits the eating of grains, legumes, processed sugar, and most sources of dairy.

The main foods allowed on a Paleo Diet are meat and fish, eggs, nuts and seeds, fruits, vegetables, and selected fats and oils such as coconut oil, olive oil or avocado oil , organic coconut oil, grass-fed butter, and grass-fed ghee. Also sweeteners in their most natural form such as honey, maple syrup, coconut sugar, and raw stevia.

The Ketogenic Diet is one that puts your body in a metabolic state where it uses the calories from fat instead of carbs for energy. Protein is limited to 20 to 30% of your diet, whereas fat would make up the balance, with only a small percentage of carbohydrates allowed in the 5 to 10% range.

Both diets eliminate grains and legumes, including corn (a grain), which is one of the most abused crops on our planet. Other than wheat, there is probably no other crop grown by farmers that is more manipulated by the use of glyphosate, which is used on a regular basis to discourage pests and in the ripening of many grains and fruits. There is much public discussion now about the toxicity of Glyphosate , but the subject is too wide ranging to dissemble here other than to say that crops with which it has been treated are best avoided by those attempting to overcome serious health issues and those trying to maximally fine-tune their diet.

Probably one of the most perfect foods for both Paleo and Ketogenic Diets are avocados. They are rich in fats and proteins and multiple other nutrients. Since they are technically a fruit, that is definitely Paleo. And their high percentage of good fats make them a perfect addition to anyone's Keto Diet.

And again, try to stick to organically sourced produce.

PURSUING A PALEO/KETO LIFESTYLE

For quite a few years now, the Paleo Diet and the Ketogenic Diet have been the major choices for healthy eating and is experiencing quite a popularity upswing. The Paleo diet is essentially based on the fact that early man was a hunter and a grazer so that basically rules out all legumes and grains which are deemed to be unnatural for our digestive systems.

The popularity of Ketogenic Diet came about by the discovery that you could lose weight more efficiently or stabilize weight when your body was in a constant state of ketosis, which is a state where your body is in an accelerated state of metabolism, constantly producing ketones.

So, if you're concerned about losing weight or you have a condition where you're trying to reduce the brown fat around your major organs, these eating plans can be very beneficial. This can be accomplished by getting your carbohydrate intake down to generally 50 grams or less per day, eliminating all processed foods from your diet; including soda, sugar, and fruit juice. However, people who have been on the SAD for many years quite often find it difficult to get into ketosis, and that's why there's been a copious number of products enabling people to accelerate into ketosis in a matter of minutes.

Personally, I have used Keto 1 with a lot of success. However, as I've gotten down to a lower percentage of body fat, I've discovered this product needs to be used with extreme care. It's like rocket fuel: there is caffeine bound to other amino acids that give you an instant boost that will power you through many hours. An added benefit will be that mental clarity and focus are extremely increased which is one of the reasons I continue to take it.

However, if you're looking to lose major weight, this is the way to go. Some people are sensitive to it, so don't be afraid to reduce the amount as you go along. I use a quarter to a half a scoop per day at this point in the morning and that works fine for me.

If you are just starting your KETO journey, this is the one! https://amzn.to/2IxvviI

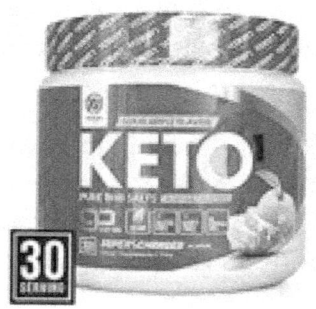

SUPER COFFEE

A number of years ago, bio-hacker Dave Asprey came up with Bulletproof Coffee. A mixture of brewed coffee, MCT coconut oil, and grass-fed butter. You really need to try this because if you really want to become lean and mean and really get down and burn off all that brown fat around your organs, this will send you on your way.

I've been starting my mornings off with this brew for a few years now, and I'll tell you the results are amazing, particularly if you combine it with any kind of a sensible diet.

Here again, as with anything, consistency is the key.

Now, if putting butter in your coffee sounds crazy there was only one kind of butter you should put in your coffee, and that's grass-fed butter. The reason you need to use grass-fed butter is that most cows are grain-fed because it's cheaper. However, cows were never really meant to be fed grain, and they can't really digest it properly. Plus, their milk will produce the kinds of fats that you don't want in your body.

Grass-fed butter has the proper ingredients that regulate cholesterol, not contribute to it. It has the best range of omega 6 to omega-3 fatty acids which actually reduce body fat. It's also a good source of vitamin K which most people today are lacking because it only gets absorbed under the right circumstances. It's also high in CLA conjugated linoleic acid, which reduces body fat mass, especially in overweight people.

Add in several tablespoons of MCT oil, the medium chain triglyceride version of coconut oil, and you have a morning drink that will supercharge you mentally and physically and rocket you into a state of ketosis for literally 4-6 hours.

This is a high-performance brew and breakfast replacement that will keep you going until lunchtime.
The recipe is:

12 oz. of the best coffee you can find
3 tbsp of MCT oil
2 tbsp grass-fed butter
Stevia to sweeten if you need

EAT YOUR SALAD

If you are like most people, you grew up hearing 'eat your vegetables.' Now that you're all grown up and have a side salad or a chef salad or chicken ranch or Caesar salad for lunch or dinner, and you think you are covering the bases veggie wise ... whoa! Think again. But wait, you say! I take a multi-vitamin! Geez!

There are a lot of issues in play here. I believe many of you have gone beyond the elementary approach dietary-wise as described above.

The real issue is we need concentrated nutrients in their most bio-available form. Preferably fresh, organic, and super green, so we can infuse as much live enzyme chlorophyll into our cells as possible.

There is nothing else but home-grown wheatgrass that fills the bill in this respect. Because it is easily grown by everyone, who has access to seeds, soil, and a place for growing with indirect sunlight.

Easy step by step instructions are in the next chapter. Believe me, whatever your misgivings may be, they are totally unfounded. And the results are beyond anything you have ever experienced!

WHEATGRASS CHLORO-PHYLL ADVENTURE

When I finally got going drinking fresh-squeezed wheatgrass juice every morning, I found out how important chlorophyll could be in my life. I had ordered a kit from the internet, and it sat under my bed for months before I finally worked up the initiative to get started doing it. I knew it was going to be a key element in my recovery, but I was still hesitant as I knew it was going to be a lot of work. And it was. But it was a daily habit that I had to just develop. But it was so worth it.

All the talk and advising by me cannot convey the experience of consuming this living nutrition directly into your body. When the grass is cut immediately before juicing you are getting the freshest live enzymes directly into your system. It's definitely a rush that most people are not prepared for. The detoxifying effects that immediately start to take place will make most people nauseous. After several days this reaction will lessen or disappear, depending on the individual circumstance. For the beginner, it is always better to mix in some organic celery and juice that behind the wheatgrass. Even so, for some, it may be difficult to tolerate. I know some of you we'll not be able to get over the hurdle of drinking a concentrated green liquid. If that's the case, you need to move on to the next chapter of powders and tablets. Although, I must tell you that none of them come close to the nutritive and rehabilitative power of freshly squeezed wheatgrass juice.

Getting started took a bit of a time commitment, but once I persisted, it didn't take much time, and like many things, eventually, it became second-nature.

Note: for juicing of wheatgrass in particular, you will need a single auger, slow masticating juicer. Nothing else will do. Just so you have an idea of what you're looking for in terms of the juicer... Omega is a reasonably priced juicer, which I have used for many years. You can find it here..

https://amzn.to/2DyhRbU

More Energy

Quite simply, fatigue Is caused by a poor diet. Once I started drinking wheatgrass juice freshly squeezed, my energy level went through the roof. Whereas the common opinion is that a person needs 8 to 10 hours of sleep, I can get by in 5 to 6.

See 'my electrical charge for photosynthesis crash course ' and supercharge yourself with the energy to power through each day.

The Lungs of the Earth

Ann Wigmore was the "Goddess" of Wheatgrass and used to say 'plants are the lungs of the earth.' With all the pollution we are surrounded with in our modern world, what a shame it is that food that is grown in the outside environment is tainted with all the chemicals from the companies who only seek to make money off their production. That is why it only makes sense to grow your own wheatgrass and other vegetables when possible.

Wheatgrass is Life's Electricity

Freshly squeezed wheatgrass juice has live enzymes which are critical for its energy giving ability. For years, scientists gave enzymes only passing credit, but now they've come to realize that they are the key catalyst and electrical force of life-energy itself. From the thinking process of your brain to digestion, to detoxification... all these processes require the activity of millions of enzymes.

Wheatgrass Builds Red Blood Cells

"Wheatgrass contains liquid oxygen," said Ann Wigmore in her revolutionary book *Wheatgrass*, first published in 1909. That was pretty heady stuff for back then when nutritional science was in its infancy. Oxygen is imperative to every bodily process. The brain uses 25% of the available oxygen in a person's body. It is no wonder then if one's diet is not at optimal levels, then they would not be surprised to be fatigued on a daily basis.

Many experiments have been done to show the widespread affliction of anemia, particularly in women. Men seem to suffer from anemia later in life, usually after age 50. It's no wonder with our modern diet, so high in starches and carbohydrates (meat and potatoes), that modern-day folks are lacking the key minerals and vitamins necessary to maintain health and vitality. The vitamins B12 and folic acid, the minerals, iron, copper, potassium, magnesium, and essential proteins are not found in abundance and in a readily accessible form compared to the intake of fresh wheatgrass juice. The above vitamins originally absorbed through the intake of fresh wheatgrass juice compared to The Standard American Diet (SAD) are essential for building iron-rich red blood cells and in turn, a body which is going through every day with health and vitality, and maximum energy.

Conclusion

Like many others before me, I have experienced the amazing turnaround of my health through the daily intake of wheatgrass juice years ago. In fact, my health improved so dramatically; I began to think I was invincible. Chlorophyll and wheatgrass had increased my energy levels to such a degree that I wandered off the path that had gotten me back to a place I wasn't familiar with at all. I quickly fell back into my old habits, my meat, and potatoes diet. It wasn't before long that I was experiencing the symptoms that had got me started on the chlorophyll and wheat-grass regimen in the first place. Over the past few years, I have since rededicated myself and decided I needed to spread the word about this amazing *Chlorophyll and Wheatgrass Diet*. I guess it's my way of owning this and taking personal responsibility and accountability for my health, and perhaps the health of others. And with that said, I will explore how to implement chlorophyll and wheatgrass into your diet in numerous ways. Optimal health can seem to be inconvenient at times, but I can assure you, the results are worth it!

GROWING WHEATGRASS

Soaking and Germinating Wheatgrass Seeds

When you think about how to grow wheatgrass at home, think organic. Red hard winter wheat seeds are the best. Purchase organic seeds from a reliable source to make sure the seeds are pesticide free. You usually can find the seeds at most health food stores and online retailers who specialize in organic seeds and supplies.

Prepare the seeds for soaking. Before the seeds can be soaked and germinated, they need to be measured and rinsed. Measure out enough seeds to create a light layer on the seed tray you use to grow the grass. For a 16" x 16" tray, use about two cups of seeds. Use a colander to rinse the seeds or simply put in your Mason jar, fill with water, swish them around and dump the water out thoroughly thru the mesh top.

Soak the seeds. Soaking the seeds initiates germination. By the end of the process, the seeds will have sprouted small roots.

- Pour cold water, preferably filtered, into the bowl of seeds. Add about three times as much water as you have seeds. Cover the bowl with a lid or plastic wrap and place it on the counter to soak for about 10 hours, or overnight.

- Drain the water from the seeds and replace it with more cold, filtered water – again, about three times as much water as you have seeds. Let it soak for another 10 hours.

- Repeat the process one more time, for a total of three long soaks.

- By the end of the last soak, the seeds should have

sprouted roots. This means they are ready to plant. Drain them and set them aside until you're ready to plant them.

Planting the Seeds

When preparing to plant in the seed tray, some people recommend lining the tray with paper towels. I don't. Here's why: first, it's a waste of paper-sourced materials, and second, it's very difficult to obtain paper towels that haven't been tainted with some kind of chemicals. Fill in an even one-inch layer of compost or potting soil in the special seed tray, in which you can make small holes for drainage with an ice pick, then use this type of punctured tray inside a tray with no holes, that way you get drainage plus ventilation.

- I always lay a fine coating of Azomite on the top. It 's the world's finest and most complete fertilizer, containing every mineral from A-Z.

- Use pre-moistened compost or potting soil, free of pesticides or other chemicals. It's important to use organic soil to get the most benefit from your wheatgrass.

Seed Planting

Spread the seeds evenly across the top of the soil. Just make sure to fill in any gaps and empty areas especially around the edges of the tray. Otherwise, your grass will be flopping over the sides.

- The seeds can be touching each other, but just make sure that there are not piles of seeds in one area.

- Water the tray thoroughly, a 16 oz. bottle of water should do it.

- Takes 6 sheets of newspaper and soak completely just by running under the faucet. Then lay them on top of the seeds, making sure to seal the edges firmly to keep out air and light. Cover with a small kitchen garbage bag.

- Moist seeds. The above is necessary to make the seeds stay moist, so if you notice the newspaper drying out, lift the newspaper occasionally and water the seeds if the paper appears to be drying out a bit.

- Just water sparingly.

- Once you lift the paper and see the sprouts have taken hold and you see the white tips of the new grass standing erect, remove the newspaper to prevent the seeds from sprouting under it.

- Continue watering the sprouted grass once a day.

Keep the grass out of sunlight. Find a corner where there is indirect light, and your grass will grow amazingly.

Fertilize. Mix a half teaspoonful of Azomite into a 16 oz. bottle of spring or filtered water, shake and spritz over the entire tray. Remember, you're staying organic here!

The Harvest

Getting ready to harvest. When the sprouted shoots are more mature, you can start to harvest them when they reach the height of at least 6 inches. Some people wait for the wheatgrass to "split." This means that the grass is ready for harvesting. At this point, the grass should be about six inches tall.

- After the time that you pull off the newspaper and turn your grass loose, continue with the indirect light, never direct sunlight.

Cut the wheatgrass about 1/2-1" above the soil. A sharp pair of kitchen scissors are best for cutting, not a knife.

- Although I only like to cut enough for that particular juicing session, wheatgrass will keep in the refrigerator for about a week, but it tastes the best and has the most live enzymes when it's cut right before you juice it.

- I personally only use the first cutting. However, you can keep watering the wheatgrass to produce a second crop.

- Sometimes you need to use a second crop before another tray matures, but don't expect it to be as tender and sweet as the first one. You will usually buy the trays in batches of 6, so make sure you start a new tray at least by the time your first batch starts to lift the newspaper.

- Keep it going. It takes quite a bit of wheatgrass to make a weekly allotment of wheatgrass juice. If you have decided to make wheatgrass a part of your life moving forward, you'll need to have several trays going at a time.

More at my site www.sogreenresource.com

SPROUTS! SPROUTS! SPROUTS!

Sprouts are the second most powerful food in my arsenal, and they are definitely a go-to snack/meal addition for a power pack of nutrients any time of the day. The live enzymes and wide nutrient profile make them a perfect complement to any juice cocktail or meal.

The beauty of sprouts is you can grow them at home in a mason jar on a window sill or kitchen countertop, preferably in indirect light. Which means you can grow them just about anywhere, any time of the year!

For a more in-depth nutritional profile, please check out my website here: www.sogreenresource.com

Broccoli Sprouts are some of the most nutritious, and (in a simplified analysis) also contain sulforaphane, which is a cancer-fighting amino acid great for the lungs and everything else.

Alfalfa sprouts, clover, mung bean, radish, etcetera; all of these and more are excellent sources of nutrition. Pick a flavor, soak them overnight and rinse daily . Easiest is in a mason jar with a plastic screw-on lid that you can get just about anywhere. Or you can just cut out a piece of screening that you can get at the dollar store and fit it into the Mason jar screw on cap. Easy.

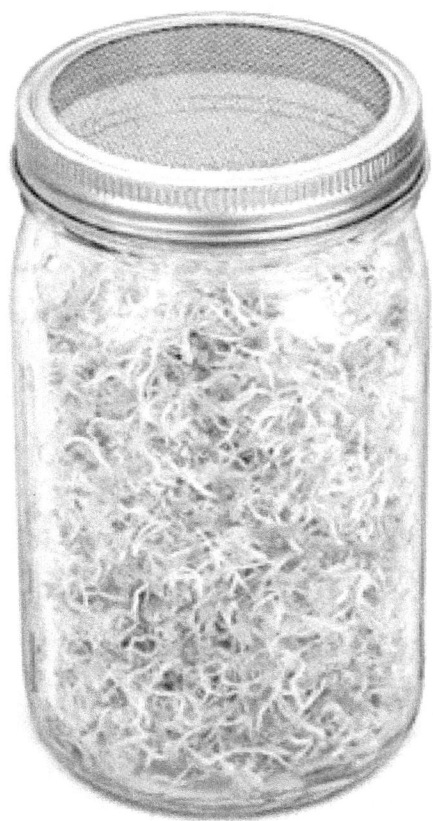

GREENS SUPPLEMENTS

Back in the day, we used to get our greens at the produce market!

Now with the proliferation of greens supplements, you can get that super nutrition in powder form, or powder compacted into pills or capsules.

Combinations of plants that have been dried and blended into a powder, green powders are designed to help you easily score an array of health-boosting vitamins and minerals. Exact ingredients vary by brand, but common ones include wheat grass, spirulina (algae), chlorella, kale, kelp, pineapple, beets, ginseng, and green tea extract. Many brands also contain pre- and probiotics as well as digestive enzymes. Mix the powder into your beverage of choice, and you're good to go.

Why Greens?

According to greens powder labels, pretty much everything can be crammed into these formulations. A lot of companies brag about improved immunity, energy levels, exercise performance, nutrient absorption, fat loss, and hormonal health.

Many common greens powder ingredients have been linked to improved exercise endurance, diabetes control, and blood stabilization. Many studies have indicated that an intake of increased greens supplements did reduce blood pressure.

In the end, the consumption of these formulations have been linked to longer, healthier lives, and greens powders are designed to help you get the vegetables and herbs you need.

However, this approach is not meant to be a substitute for vegetables in your daily diet. You need live enzymes and fiber. "Greens powders should only be used as an addition to a diet that's rich in whole foods, including fruits and vegetables. So, make sure you get a couple of servings of fresh fruits and vegetables every day."

After all, the body reacts quite differently to whole foods than it does to isolated vitamins. And while greens powders do contain many whole foods (in extract form), eating broccoli powder and beetroot extract is still very different than if you ate a plate full of broccoli or beets.

That being said, I use 2 greens supplements in combination or individually, depending on the rotation I am cycling, whether I am doing wheatgrass that day or week.

I have used many over the years, but Amazing Grass has been my favorite for quality and economy. Over the past several years, I have added Organifi, which is a unique combo of dried wheatgrass juice and select ingredients including moringa, ashwagandha, spirulina, chlorella, beets, and turmeric . . . the list goes on.

This stuff is a true SuperFood!

To be honest, this stuff has a super price for most people. This is kind of where the wheat is separated from the chaff, so to speak, when it comes to your dedication in this area. My general rule is quality and affordability, but this is obviously a different equation from individual to individual. But if you have some flexibility in your budget, this is where to go for it!

Organifi is truly a unique and superior supplement right now. If you are not taking anything besides your regular vitamin supplementation, you will probably realize measurable changes in your energy levels and sense of overall well-being.

As a final thought, Organifi is a gently dried juice, making it nutritionally superior to formulations of ground grass.

NOOTROPICS

Nootropics are kind of a catchall for drugs, supplements, and any substances that might improve cognitive functions, including creativity, memory, problem-solving, and motivation.

I have tried the following and a few more, but always start out with half the dosage and work your way up (with your doctor's approval, that is).

Great success can be had with fine-tuning. However, after all is said and done, the folks at Neurohacker have come up the ultimate daily blend in Qualia. The quality and economy can't be beaten!

1 - Caffeine - caffeine is the most widely consumed psychoactive substance in the world. It's found in coffee, cocoa, tea, guarana, and many other leafy plants. It works by blocking the Dennison receptors in your brain. The end result is that it makes you less tired. Obviously, it's habit-forming and quite addictive.

2 - L-Theanine - is a naturally occurring amino acid in a variety of teas. It actually has a calming effect and increases creativity, particularly when paired with caffeine.

3 - Bacopa Monnieri - is an herbal supplement which has been shown to improve memory and information processing when taken consistently.

4 - Rhodiola Rosea - is another herb that can help your body adjust to times of high stress and also reduce mental fatigue.

5 - Panax Ginseng - abyssal plant used for centuries in Asia as a brain stimulant and general overall body tonic.

6 - Ginkgo biloba - the leaves from the tree are said to improve memory and mental processing and also helps to reduce stress.

7 - Noopept - it's a fast-acting synthetic that is said to improve memory; however more research is probably needed on long-term use.

8 - Piracetam - another synthetic similar to Noopept in its makeup and has been shown to improve memory. Even though it is widely available and promoted as a *smart drug*, the research is not complete.

9 - Modafinil - this is a prescription drug that was originally invented in France to treat narcolepsy. It has similar properties to those of amphetamines or cocaine, yet acts on the body much differently. It is not a stimulant and thus, not addictive when taken at low dosages. That's because it's a eugeroic - a wakeful-ness-promoting agent.

10 - Adderall, Ritalin - prescription strength and stimulants. Doctor recommended. You know the deal.

NAD+ and PTEROSTILBENE

The importance of NAD+ to cellular health has been known in the scientific community for over a century. It supports DNA health, controls cellular metabolism, and regulates our "longevity" genes, which play a critical role in aging and long-term health. Shortages of NAD+ leave our cells at risk for mutation, dysfunction, degeneration, and even death. Recent studies show that levels of NAD+ decline as we age, suggesting an explanation for why we succumb to varying health issues as we get older. Replenishing NAD+ is an advanced, science-based strategy to maintain energy and staying healthy as we age. NIAGEN® is the brand name for nicotinamide riboside (NR), a naturally-occurring compound found in trace amounts in milk. Pioneered and patented by ChromaDex, Inc., NIAGEN® is now the subject of many exciting studies on topics such as glucose control, weight management, and anti-aging and has been licensed to several companies for manufacture and distribution.

Pterostilbene vs. Resveratrol

Pterostilbene has been shown to have the same antioxidant potential as resveratrol. However, pterostilbene is more fat-soluble and less susceptible to degradation; this leads to a greater half-life in the body compared to resveratrol (105 vs. 14 minutes). These specific structural differences seem to make resveratrol more adept at combating reactive oxygen species (ROS) in whole blood and lymphocytes and pterostilbene is better at targeting extra-cellular ROS.* Such extra-cellular ROS are often responsible for tissue damage with an imbalanced inflammatory response, amongst other things. As such, pterostilbene and resveratrol tend to be more complementary in their action than competitive. Work in animals has even suggested synergies between the two, along with quercetin.

NAD+ and PTEROSTILBENE INTRO

For quite a few years now I have been taking NR (NAD+ precursor) and Pterostilbene. NAD+ (nicotinamide adenine dinucleotide) is a coenzyme found in all living cells, and it's required for the intracellular biological processes that make life possible. Processes include converting nutrients into energy, supporting the health of DNA, and controlling circadian rhythms.

Pterostilbene closely resembles resveratrol on a molecular level, but it is 4 times more potent, and its bioavailability is far superior. It is called a sirtuin activator.

QUALIA – THE FUTURE OF NOOTROPICS

Qualia is a supplement that is based on the idea that the body has an innate ability that can be supported and enhanced for creating its own health system. It's a whole system approach to supplying the body and the brain with the herbs and micronutrients necessary to stimulate optimum health.

This has been my go-to supplement and actually my main vita-min, and herbal nootropics supplement for the past several years right after they came out with it.

The ingredients of Qualia Mind below:

Supplement Facts

Serving Size: 7 Vegetarian Capsules
Servings Per Container: 22

	Amount	%DV		Amount	%DV
Vitamin C (as ascorbic acid)	100 mg	111%	Alpha-Glyceryl Phosphoryl Choline (alpha-GPC)	200 mg	**
Vitamin D3 (as cholecalciferol)	25 mcg (1,000 IU)	125%	DHA (as Docosahexaenoic Acid from Algae)	200 mg	**
Niacin (as niacinamide)	50 mg	313%	Cognizin® Citicoline	150 mg	**
Vitamin B6 (as pyridoxal 5'-phosphate)	20 mg	1176%	Bacopamine	100 mg	**
Vitamin B12 (as methylcobalamin)	1000 mcg	41667%	Mucuna pruriens Seed Extract (50% L-Dopa)	100 mg	**
Pantothenic Acid (as calcium pantothenate)	50 mg	1000%	Phosphatidylserine (Sharp-PS® Green) (from sunflower lecithin)	100 mg	**
Acetyl-L-Carnitine HCL	500 mg	**	Theobromine	100 mg	**
Artichoke Stem and Leaf Extract (5% cynarin)	500 mg	**	Anhydrous Caffeine	90 mg	**
Bacopa monnieri Leaf Extract (45% bacosides)	300 mg	**	Celastrus paniculatus Seed Extract	60 mg	**
Rhodiola rosea Root (3% rosavins; 1% salidrosides)	300 mg	**	Ginkgo biloba Leaf Extract (24% glycosides)	50 mg	**
DL-Phenylalanine	300 mg	**	Coleus forskohlii Root Extract (20% forskolin)	20 mg	**
Uridine-5'-Monophosphate (disodium)	250 mg	**	Pyrroloquinoline Quinone	10 mg	**
N-Acetyl-L-Tyrosine	250 mg	**	Huperzine A (Huperzia serrata leaf standardized extract)	50 mcg	**
Taurine	200 mg	**			
L-Theanine	200 mg	**			

** Daily Value (DV) not established

** Daily Value (DV) not established

You can check out the particulars here.
www.neurohacker.com
Get a 15% discount with the coupon code GARY123 .

HERBS

Aside from herbs that you might use in your kitchen, here are some herbs of the medicinal variety or what we would be concerned with the most here.

From my experience goldenseal and olive leaf, and damiana leaf are the most effective antimicrobial herbs to keep you out of the doctor's office. If I ever get a sign of a sore throat or am feeling a bit off, I take a few of each before bed or every few hours throughout the day to kill off whatever.

TONIC EXTRACTS

Going on 5 years now I have been taking various herbal and tonic extracts made by a company called Tonic Tinctures. Their passion for quality and excellence in their formulations has caused me to never look elsewhere. I do not receive any kickback here but just have to mention them as one of the primary members of my Combination of Things Club.

Whether it's extracted from berries, mushrooms, or roots and leaves, they all have something valuable to offer and when the nutrient profile is presented this way it's from the whole plant. Except, for example, ginseng, where the root is the part that has the most to offer.

I have been taking most of the items described below for many years with fantastic results, both short-term and long-term. Again, there are no specific health claims made here for any specific conditions and always consult with your healthcare provider before taking any of these supplements or embarking upon any exercise programs recommended in this book. That being said, there's a reason these supplements are so available and popular, but you have to judge for yourself. Some work better than others on an individual basis. Essentially, it's trying a brand or certain supplement to find one that really works for you.

I discovered Tonic Tinctures, www.tonictinctures.com over 5 years ago and haven't found any other company producing extracts anywhere near the quality that this company produces. Here again, I receive no compensation for recommending them, I'm just spreading the word.

They have evolved over years and years of experimentation to a multi-extraction process that yields the purest and most concentrated extracts I've ever taken.

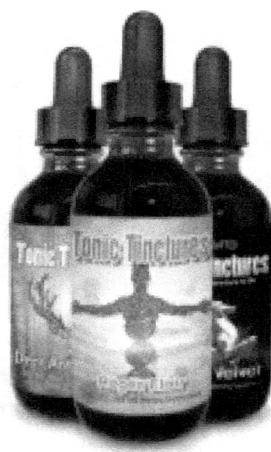

Tonic Tincture Power Pack Liquid Extract

DEER ANTLER VELVET

Throughout human history, people of all ages in Asia have been using dealer deer antler velvet isotonic and revitalizer. It supplies igf-1 and stimulates the endocrine glands.

As with all good tonics it needs to be cycled and watched carefully to avoid overuse. Although I've never had a problem in all the years that I've been using it.

PANAX GINSENG

Likewise, ginseng has many fantastic benefits as it has also been used in Asia for centuries as a general tonic and healer of many ills.

I have been using the same brand for over 30 years and would never think of using anything else as my mainstay tonic for daily use as the quality has never wavered. In this age of one-hit wonders, you never know with you can depend from one batch to the next on the quality of the formulation. Of course, the company I'm talking about is Ilwha, and again I get no compensation for boosting them, and there's also been much controversy throughout the years concerning the fact that Reverend Moon had started it and has owned the company since its origination.

That being said, I have never found a ginseng product that's been made with its unique cold process while maintaining continuing quality to this day.

When I am not taking this on a daily basis, my body lets me know. Highly recommended. I also use Tonic Tinctures Panax ginseng extract as a supplement, and it is excellent.

REISHI, CHAGA MUSHROOM

Great for immune system, adrenal, stress, cognition, stamina regeneration, and again general tonic.

CORDYCEPS MUSHROOM

Great for cleansing the lungs, stamina, intimacy, immune system building, you name it, it's the best.

LION'S MANE MUSHROOM

Great for hormone stabilization and stamina.

BLACK ANT

The supplement of Emperors since the beginning of time; it's been taken for strength and stamina. Be an Ant! - strong, quick thinking, and powerful for your size!

GOJI BERRY

Very high in vitamin c and antioxidants.

ASHWAGANDHA

General tonic and stress management.

ASTRALAGUS

Antioxidant strength and power for better breathing, immunity, and overall tonic.

THE EXERCISES

THE DAILY 1 2 3

This is my morning exercise thing. It takes 10 minutes.
It's quick and easy. The emphasis is on core strength and back and hamstring stretch. These are key elements for me since my accident because I am always tight in the lower back and hamstrings. Also, if you don't exercise daily and sit most of the time like most people, YOU NEED TO DO THIS!

1. Touch toes or hang there without forcing it until you start to unfold.

2. Then sit on a mat or carpet and do 20 sit-ups or more, if comfortable, with your knees up.

3. Next, lying with your back flat on the floor with legs straight, raise your legs slowly in 30-degree increments pausing for the count of ten until your legs are at 90 degrees.

4. Then, bring your legs back over your head, rotating at the hips only until your toes touch the floor behind your head. Keep your legs straight. If you are new, this will be difficult. Hold the position until the count of 20.

When I started out years ago, this took several days but gradually your body will establish a memory, and this will feel normal and comfortable. This is called the Plough posture in yoga.

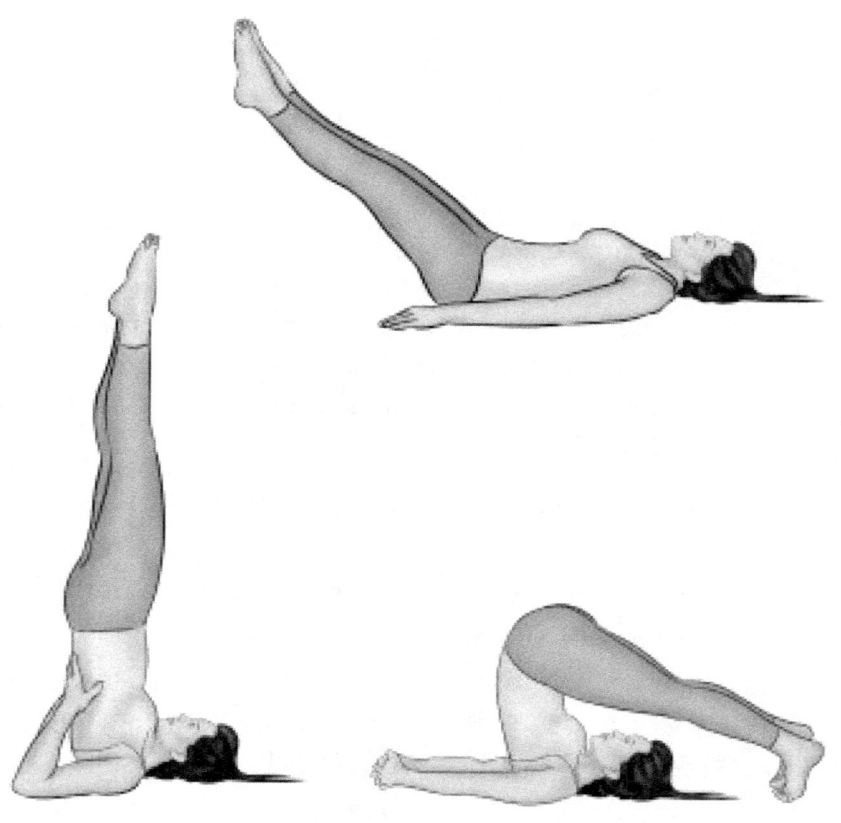

5. Now, slowly raise your legs and at the same time move your hands to your lower back, pushing lightly and pointing your toes toward the sky until your entire weight is on your shoulders. Voila! You're doing a shoulder stand and the inversion portion of your mini work-out. Hold this upright position until the count of 100 or more.

6. Then, once again bring your legs back down over your head to return your toes to the floor behind your head. the stretch should be easier this time due to the change in blood flow. Hold to a count of at least 20 or more until the tension is released.

7. Return your legs to a 90 degree angle, then 45 degree holding each phase for the count of ten .. then to the floor.

8. Relax .. Dead Man pose

9. Turn over onto your stomach, placing your hands beneath your shoulders in push up position. Raise your head as you gently assist the raising of your entire chest as far as you are able. Do not tense or involve your lower half or legs. This pose is to condition the spine and lower back as well as the organs of the lower chest. Just excellent ! After repeating this 3 times slowly, push up to a sitting position sitting on your heels. At first this may be uncomfortable, but is a great stretch for the legs and feet.

Refer to next illustration >

10. Next, lower your chest down onto your thighs, face on the floor with arms down grasping your heels. Hold.

11. Slowly raise to a standing position, bringing your hands up from your sides in a circular motion above your head while inhaling deeply, hold and then bring them down while exhaling completely. Voila !

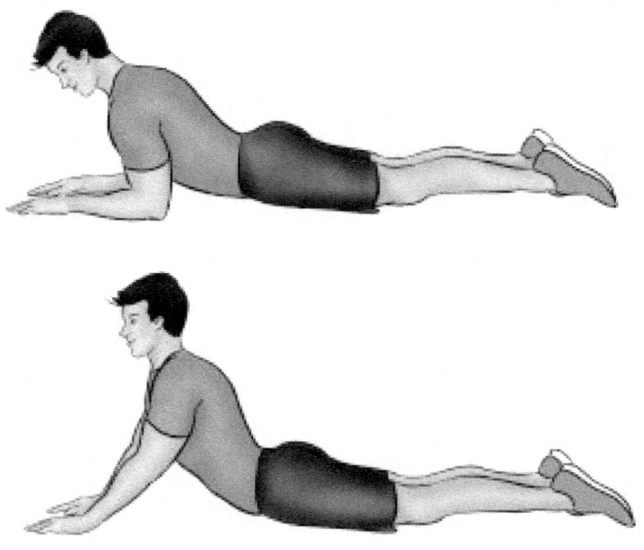

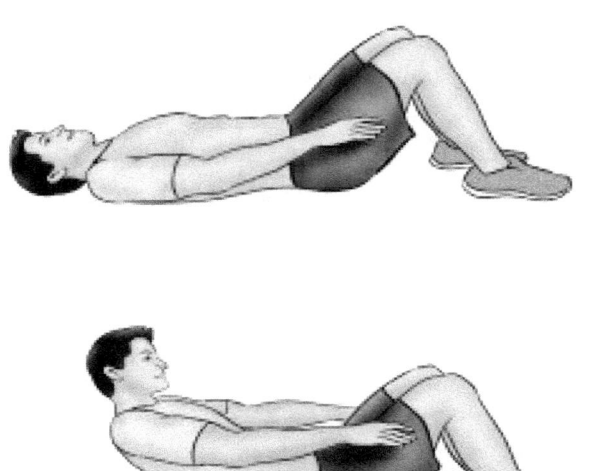

Reversing gravity and achieving balance

It's a fact. We spend most of our time right-side up. As a result, we end up looking like various degrees of the illustration below.

From the time we are born gravity keeps us grounded. We can only escape as far as our own muscles will take us or perhaps higher with artificial means such as airplanes or more portable flying devices. It is constantly pulling us toward the center of our planet. Our organs are being pulled earthbound as well as our blood, cells, etc. Everything, anything with a mass within us and around us is being pulled downward. This constant gravitational downward pull, along with general everyday movement is what get your discs between your lumbar vertebrae looking like squashed mushroom caps instead of the squared off sponges they started out as illustrated below.

Also, the constant pressure squeezes the moisture out of your disks like a sponge that's been wrung out. When your disks are being constantly squeezed, they can't draw in the necessary moisture they need to revitalize themselves and remain healthy. Only by separating the vertebrae can this occur.

The most efficient way to do this is to stretch the spine.

GRAVITY

So, of course, gravity is omnipresent in our lives. Our challenge is to figure out how to turn it to our advantage through inversion. I feel as though I have found that way in regards to the rehabilitation of my broken back. I have found it true that through inversion, the increased blood flow going to the discs between my vertebrae has rehabilitated them. There is no doubt that the traction-like stretching effect increases the blood flow to the sponge-like discs, which are aching for nourishment.

This is not a one-time treatment. A daily routine is definitely necessary. The human body responds to daily routine and nourishment.

And since circulatory issues have been increasingly prevalent for an aging population, I feel that inversion can't help but cure a lot of issues in this area through essentially backflushing your system for a few minutes a day, every day, by hanging upside down. By doing this, you are reversing the normal flow of blood throughout your body.

Others have noted that monkeys and sloths hang upside down so they must've known something we didn't. However, they don't hang upside down for health reasons. Many times, it's a matter of convenience, shielding themselves from enemies, or in the case of bats, the fact that they can't take off from an upright position, hanging upside down gives them a head start regarding flight.

A bar with gravity boots is easiest if you are in relatively good shape. However, if not, you can use a different type of inversion equipment called a Teeter Inversion Table which requires no

Gary S. Patterson

boots.

YOGA HEAD STAND

Many years before I had my motorcycle accident I used to practice headstands daily.

You can achieve and enjoy all the benefits of the hanging type inversion, except for the stretching. It is usually recommended before learning and practising the headstand that you are free from neck and spinal issues.

Even these days, if I'm on the road I will still include it in my routine. At least a shoulder stand, which is less apt to aggravate any lower back issues (as illustrated earlier).

You are still giving your organs a nice reverse flush to all organs, adrenals, etc.

Also, fluids are drained from the feet and legs as a great preventative for the dreaded varicose veins.

TYPES OF INVERSION

Gravity Boots

This was my first choice as I've always been an athletic type and was in reasonably good shape. I would only recommend this for people who feel reasonably confident in their abilities. It is also going to offer you the maximum stretch and traction like separation of the vertebrae to facilitate maximum blood flow to the discs, or, what may have remained of them in my case. Remember, your discs are like sponges, and to remain healthy, and in my case regenerate, they need space to ensure the maximum amount of fluid being allowed to circulate around the discs. Obviously, the range of exercises is greater and offers a greater variety in the 180-degree position.

It is possible to execute rudimentary exercises on a slant board or inversion table at angles greater than 90 degrees. However, the number of exercises possible will be greater when in full 180-degree inversion.

Gravity   Boots   with   180-degree   inversion

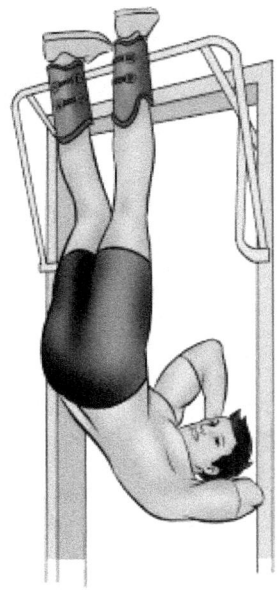

Teeter   Inversion   Table

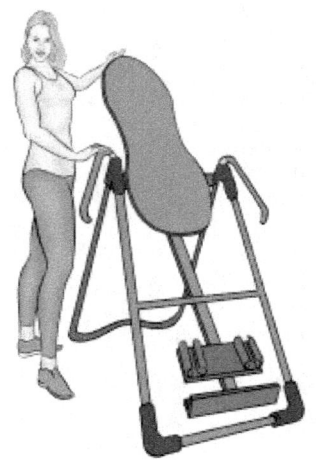

Inverted Position

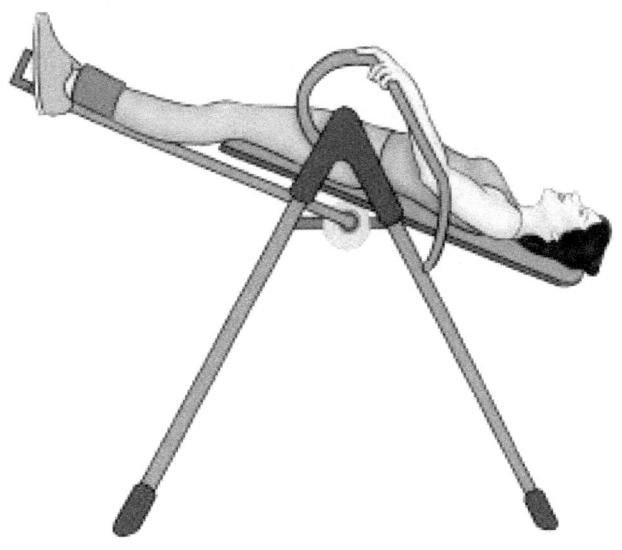

YOGA

Yoga, what is there to say about it. It's an all-encompassing system for fine-tuning your body and your mind. If time permits, it can quickly become a part of your daily lifestyle. As I am not promoting yoga as a lifestyle and just a solution to several issues addressed in this book, I am presenting several poses that are not time-consuming and easy to do.

Specifically, these are core strengthening, and hip opening type poses, offering variety and quick results. However, they must be practiced regularly in order to continue producing benefits.

Different   positions   with   yoga

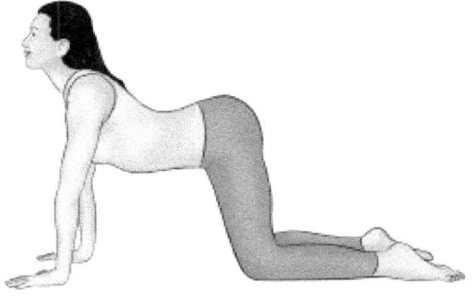

Stretching is the best form of Yoga to loosen up and strengthen the body.

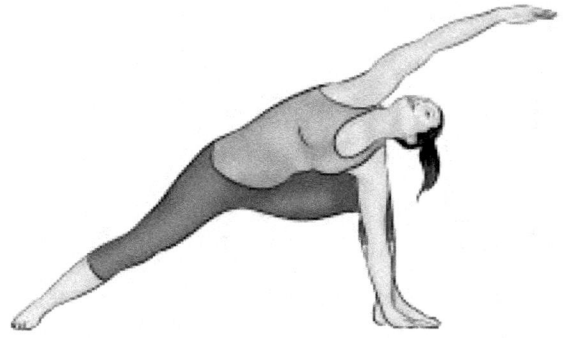

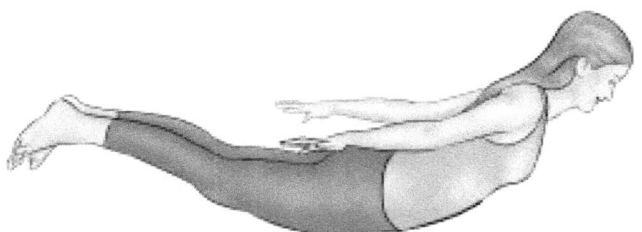

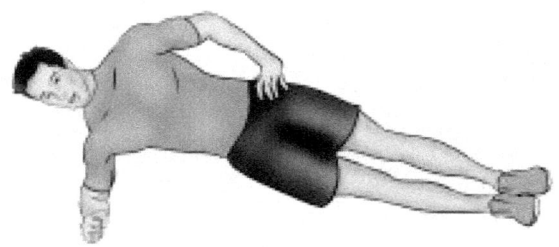

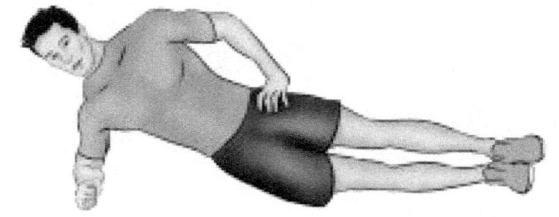

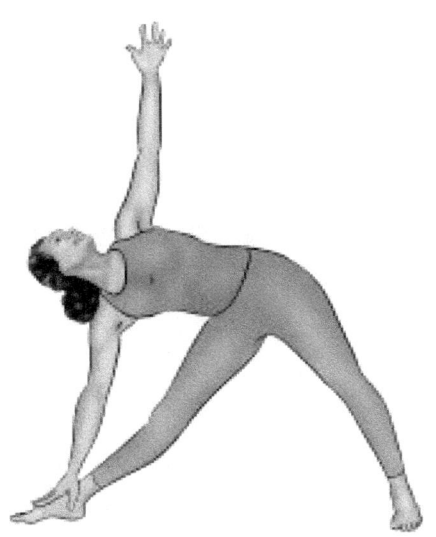

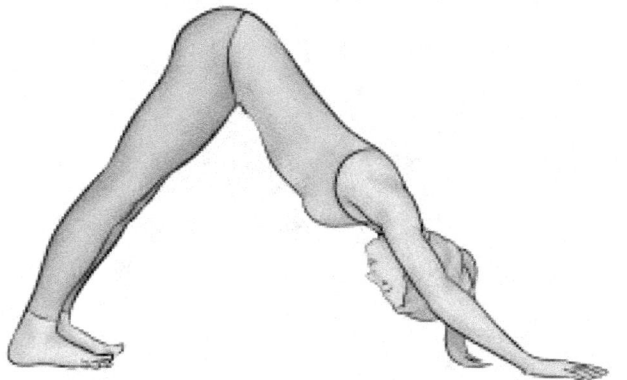

WALKING IS THE BEST

Walking is the best because it's easy and natural. The benefits of simple even paced walking are many to your health and longevity.

1. Going outside and taking a walk automatically lifts your mood and supports your immune system, because, no matter the weather, you must walk. What's the alternative? Sitting in a chair in the house? And when I say walk, I mean walk like you're going somewhere with a purpose; full stride and arms are swinging or pumping. No window-shopping stroll for us! Always go with a plan for a prescribed route or Point A to point B, including a time-frame for finishing so that you will have a sense of accomplishment when done.

2. Walk and stimulate creativity. Solutions to problems often appear when you are not thinking about them and instead of watching clouds or talking to birds.

3. Your metabolism is directly stimulated by how fast or slow you walk or run. Try sprinting a short distance and then walking and repeat. This is how our ancestors moved. Fight or flight. It's the natural way we were built.

4. Walking is motion and the more motion you have; the more your cells are stimulated.

5. Walking at least 30 minutes at a time can, over time, stabilize weight, help you lose weight, lower blood pres-

sure, and generally improve all those health markers that are your doctor's concerns. However, you've got to be proactive about scheduling your activity on a daily basis.

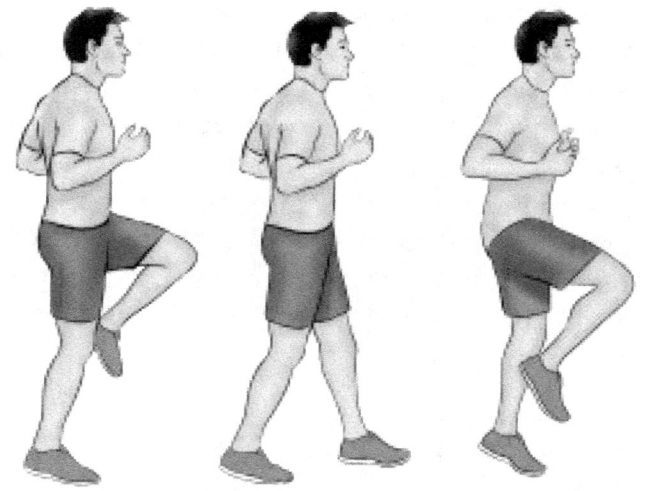

HIIT

High-Intensity Interval Training

It's a form of interval training and cardiovascular exercise in one incorporating short periods of intense anaerobic exercise with less intense recovery times. There are beginner and advanced stages with this type of training as with anything. Naturally, some people will take it to the max. For our purposes, we're going to assume that you're in moderate shape and ambulatory at the least. (Haha.)

I do this quite a bit, and it's the most basic form of interval training. Start out with a brisk walk to warm up and after your feeling loosened up, break into a moderate sprint for as long as you're comfortable with then back to walking. Keep doing this until you're tired or until you've covered your predetermined distance for the day. Mine is usually three to four miles or a 35- to 45-minute workout. This is the amount of time that you really need for your body to reap the benefits of your activity.

Here again, we're just trying to begin to increase our cardiovascular activity here, we're not training for the Olympics, so take it easy when first starting out.

The combination of things is like a biorhythm. With a HIIT workout, it's a give and take situation, hard and relaxed, nutrition and food, then exercise.

It's HRV, heart rate variability, fast and slow; it's not just one straight-ahead monolithic approach.
Your body, as well as your mind, will become bored with a

straight-ahead, everyday approach to both eating and exercising with the same technique and principles. You have to change it up and vary it.

Essentially, it's the formula of work. Exertion, pause, rest, exertion, pause, rest, exertion, pause, rest.

The Nitric Oxide Dump

Dr. Zach Bush has come up with the ultimate compact exercise routine for releasing that beneficial nitric oxide that permeates your entire body.

It takes just 4 minutes and requires no equipment or fancy outfits.

See the following page for illustrations of these simple exercises.

1ST – STANDING SQUATS – 10 REPS EACH X 4

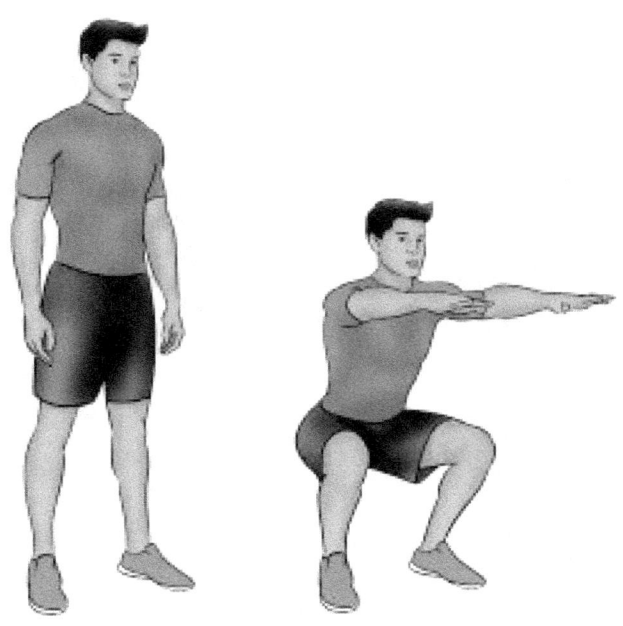

2ND - ARM RAISES - 10 REPS EACH X 4

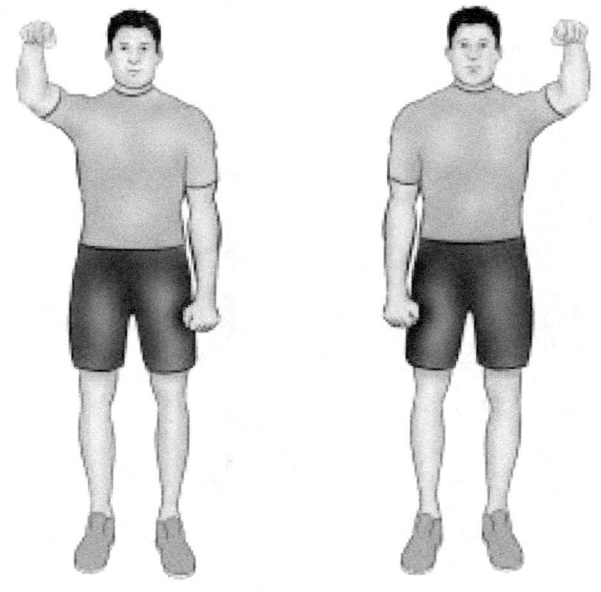

3RD - STATIONARY JACKS -
10 REPS EACH X 4

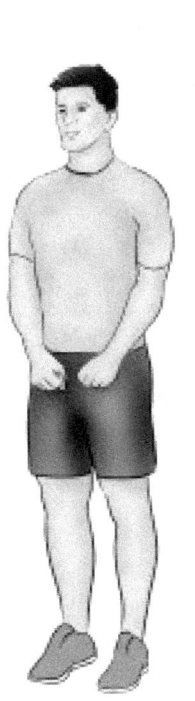

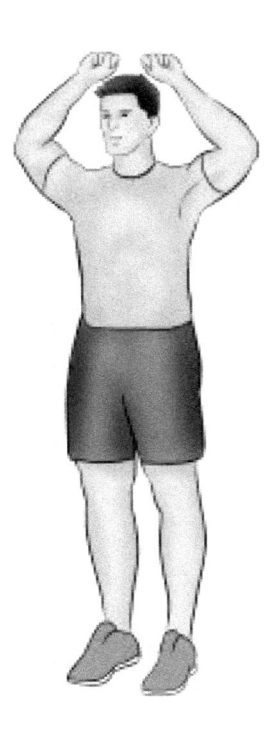

4TH - ARM PRESS - 10 REPS EACH X 4

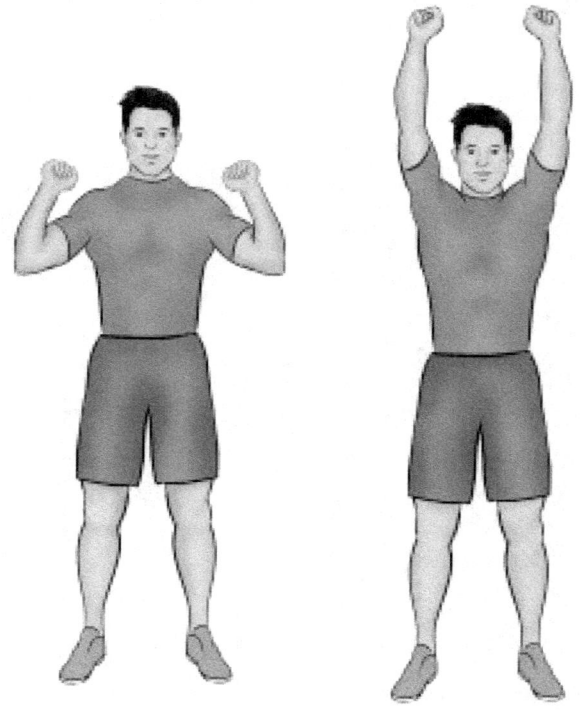

MEDITATION

When I was living in Venice, CA in the late 60s, a friend recommended a meditation instructor and one day we went and received our mantras and instructions. My counselor received my mantra by placing his hands on the back of my neck. He then wrote it on a blackboard. He proceeded to instruct me on how to pronounce this Greek-like multisyllabic word. Placing emphasis on certain syllables, but most importantly to let it flow and not dwell on the mantra itself. This was all given with sincerity and tempered earnestness. That convinced me this meditation thing might have something going for it.

I returned to my room to practice with the technique I had been given and soon had moved beyond my body. I could actually look down upon myself sitting there. After an undetermined amount of time, I came back down to earth, so to speak, and was amazed. Needless to say, I was hooked.

To this day, I find a quiet spot, and for a few minutes every day, I leave the daily grind and find my private space.

QIGONG

This is a description from Wikipedia... I contribute monthly and would encourage you to do so as well. It is an invaluable resource and treasure.

"Qigong is a holistic system of coordinated body posture and movement, breathing, and meditation used for the purposes of health, spirituality, and martial arts training. With roots in Chinese medicine, philosophy, and martial arts, qigong is traditionally viewed as a practice to cultivate and balance qi (chi), translated as "life energy."[3]

Qigong practice typically involves moving meditation, coordinating slow flowing movement, deep rhythmic breathing, and calm, meditative state of mind. Qigong is now practiced throughout China and worldwide for recreation, exercise and relaxation, preventive medicine and self-healing, alternative medicine, meditation and self-cultivation, and training for martial arts.

Qigong comprises a diverse set of practices that coordinate body (調身), breath (調息), and mind (調心) based on Chinese philosophy.[27][28] Practices include moving and still meditation, massage, chanting, sound meditation, and non-contact treatments, performed in a broad array of body postures. Qigong is commonly classified into two foundational categories: 1) dynamic or active qigong (dong gong), with slow flowing movement; and 2) meditative or passive qigong (jing gong), with still positions and inner movement of the breath.[29]:21770–21772

From a therapeutic perspective, qigong can be classified into two systems: 1) internal qigong, which focuses on self-care and self-cultivation; and 2) external qigong, which involves treatment by a therapist who directs or transmits qi.[29]:21777–21781

As moving meditation, qigong practice typically coordinates slow, stylized movement, deep diaphragmatic breathing, and calm mental focus, with visualization of guiding qi through the body. While implementation details vary, generally qigong forms can be characterized as a mix of four types of practice: dynamic, static, meditative, and activities requiring external aids.

I have incorporated Qigong meditation techniques on a basic level into my meditative time over the past several years.

To be sure, Qigong is a complex practice that is worthy of a time investment that many people will find too demanding, but I believe a steady application of even its most basic precepts and practices can be extremely rewarding. I know they have for me.

I encourage everyone to give it a try. It is amazing the life energy within us just waiting to be activated.

This is the book that got me started –
The Way of Energy by Master Lam Kam Chuen introducing the Zhan Zhuang system of "Standing Like a Tree." https://amz-n.to/2WXp7p4

I started standing and caught on right away. I had meditated in the past, but this is a release of energy that is surprising at first. It's a commitment that I would imagine is difficult for some to maintain. It was for me. As I write this, I am returning to re-commit since I miss the sense of control and confidence I experienced by simply learning to stand as instructed. This represents to me how simple and direct our energy connection is to the world around and within us.

COLD SHOWERS

When I first started finishing my morning showers off with a cold rinse of about 10 to 20 seconds, I thought I was onto something.

I just thought it was invigorating and maybe helping to build my immune system.

It wasn't until I accidentally read something about cold showers being a daily therapy that I started to take them seriously.

It's kind of one of those things that you know, but it's not omnipresent in your mind. Years ago I belonged to a quote-unquote health club where they had a cold pool that you could jump into after being in the sauna. A lot of guys couldn't do it, but I always enjoyed it. And of course, there were the Nordic countries with the traditions of the ice pools, ice baths, jumping into snow banks, etc. So, I just gradually started to stretch the cold shower part out longer, gradually stretching it out longer every time until I couldn't stand it anymore.

Eventually, the water wasn't cold enough, although in the winter months you will find that the groundwater going through your home water system is much colder. If you are a morning shower person and on-the-clock, in the winter you will doing yourself some real immune and inflammatory response boosting if you can hold your cold shower for a count of at least 60 seconds after turning off the hot water portion of your shower. Wow!

BREATHING BASICS

Of all the years that I visited doctors regarding my asthma, no one ever suggested that I should do breathing exercises or breathe in a particular way. As a child, I never questioned that approach. Children have so many different concerns ping-ponging around in their head; that's the least of their concerns to question what the doctor's telling you. Haha, that comes later in adulthood.

My father continually asked if I was catching flies! Heh, that's how I breathed. No-one EVER said there was a reason to breathe through your nose. I mean, how was it possible that my doctors didn't know about Butyenko's discoveries in breathing techniques in 1950, some of which had been practiced by yogis for like forever?

The 8 Hour Sleep Paradox in 2015 is a very comprehensive read on why proper breathing during sleep affects us so profoundly since, hey, we spend 1/3 of our life screwing up our health if we're snoring our nights away.

The inner cavities of your nose and sinuses are designed to swirl the in-going air in a spinning turbo-like fashion, which in turn, out creates nitric oxide. Wow! Can't get enough of that! Its main effect is that of
vasodilation, so if you're a mouth breather, chances are you've got sinus issues. Heady stuff? (Pardon the pun!)

In this search is where I discovered mouth-taping. You want to get the micro-pore surgical tape and tape your mouth shut before going to sleep. Initially, I was a bit apprehensive, being asthmatic. What if I stopped breathing? Or couldn't get any or enough air? Didn't happen. The very first morning I awoke more easily and refreshed. I am not saying it was a brand-new world, but I could feel the difference. When you breathe through your nose, the inner chambers of your nose swirl the air and create nitric oxide is what I had read. Nitric oxide is energizing and evidently, that night long process did the trick. Wow! How about every night? This was looking like a serious endeavor. So, I did it, and my health has been improving steadily. Now, mind you, I am doing multiple 'protocols,' so this had to noticeable. And it was! So, this particular regimen became a keeper.

TOOLS AND DEVICES

NanoVi - To Your Health!

My friends, I am convinced that this is one of the most important medical devices ever created. By simply breathing the vapor
from the device, it carries a bio-identical signal to your cells with
good ROS (reactive oxygen species) to accelerate cell repair. This
is not only mind-boggling but also has never been done before!

This might have been a more convincing testimonial if I had
been initially skeptical. But I wasn't. I knew instantly what the
NanoVi was designed for and more importantly, what the results
could be. You see, I have been growing and juicing my own wheatgrass for many years now and thus understand the importance of
infusing live enzymes to the cells.

I have been using the NanoVi for about 2 years now.
From the first months of use, I felt an increase in my overall energy level. People who met me for the first time were amazed at
my age and youthful appearance, more so than usual.

At about the 3- or 4-month stage, I noticed a change in my BMI
that I almost couldn't believe. My body started to look more like
it did in my 20s. It's the type of thing that sounds fantastical unless you experience it.

Arthritis in my hands and elbows vanished. Poof!

Also, I didn't realize the change in HRV until I went from a brisk
walk or jog to stop and enter a qigong posture. I could immedi-

ately go to a meditative state. WOW! The recovery mechanism that was there was astounding.

I have had asthma since childhood. The breathing equation is also complicated by my smoking various substances, inhaling asbestos fibers, and a myriad of toxins in my youth. I still have to use an inhaler, depending on the weather changes that seem to be affecting me the most. But I can't help but feel that I am gaining ground on that front.

My family doctor looks at me incredulously and asks what I am doing there? A resting pulse of 54 and BP 107/87. And all I do now is a brisk walk for 30 minutes each day.

Finally, I must say that when I found the NanoVi, I was desperately looking for something that would help me clarify what I can only call 'foggy brain.' I spend a lot of time in front of the computer and in addition to the eye strain, I think the EMF exposure was accumulating.

Well, I have found that with the NanoVi I feel progressively clearer mentally every day.
You have got to try this!
www.eng3corp.com

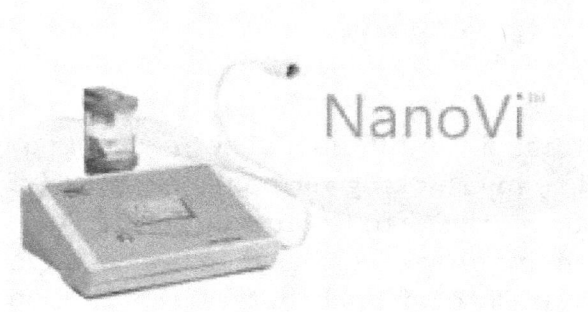

PEMF – A POSSIBLE
LIFE CHANGER

Pulsed Electromagnetic Fields is a term for a therapy that most closely resembles the bio-electric activity in our bodies cells so that they are most receptive to the exchange of energy. Although quite a few studies have been done and this entire therapeutic arena has been around for years, it has been largely ignored by the mainstream medical establishment. As I have said before, I am not listing sources bibliographically or otherwise because I believe that in this format, no one is going to pore over obscure references to papers published decades ago. But they are there if you want scientific substantiation. NASA knew and recognized all of the bio-electric activity in our cells decades ago. The scientific originator of their proprietary equipment was inventor Dr. Robert Dennis, who although not credited on the original patents, was recently verified as the original inventor leading to his updated versions, the modern ICES® DigiCeutical® technology developed in 2013-2014.

On his website, Micro-pulse.com, you will see the validity of the technology.

I have used the A9a model extensively on multiple areas of my body with a great deal of success. For example, I have dealt with a pulled hamstring and ruptured Achilles tendon for over 20 years, going through various stages of wellness in this area.

Almost immediately after beginning periods of therapy with the A9, I realized improvements in residual pain and tension with my hamstring and increased flexibility. Has healing begun? That's hard to say. Time will tell. I do know that the A9 has almost instant positive effects on my back pain and stiffness on cold winter mornings. This is a bonus since it's portable and wearable.

It's also the most affordable PEMF device available.

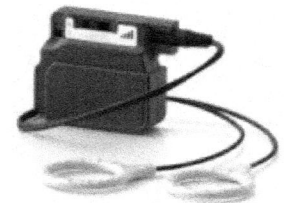

ICES® DigiCeutical® A9a

JOOVV INFRARED LIGHT

Infrared and near-infrared light therapies have been gaining in popularity in the past few years, even though they have been around for a long time.

A lot of the increase is due to advances in LED technology and at the forefront is a company named JOOVV. Through innovation and quality manufacturing, they have become the leader in LED therapy devices that others can merely imitate.

I have been using their original combo unit since right near their entering the marketplace. The combo unit comprises alternating red and near-infrared LED light bulbs and puts out energy that will change your day almost instantly.

The many proven benefits are:

1 - an increase in collagen production - collagen is the most prevalent protein in the body accounting for more than 70% being attributed to skin elasticity.

2 - a reduction in joint pain and inflammation - arthritis and injury-caused joint and tendon pain are gone!

3 - an improvement in sleep quality – this therapy helps to stabilize our circadian rhythms.

4 - augments weight loss - encourages the release of fat from the cells.

5 - speeds muscle recovery - reduction in oxidative stress is the

key.

6 - Improved physical performance – increased. <u>Aids testosterone production in men.</u>

Stay young, get young and energized with JOOVV! Get more info here - www.joovv.com

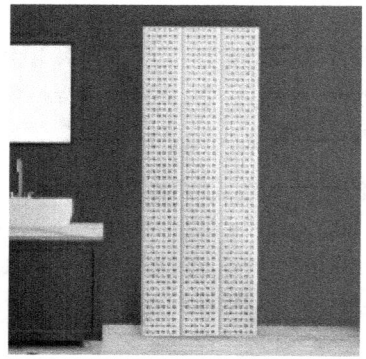

JOOVV Elite Wall Set-up

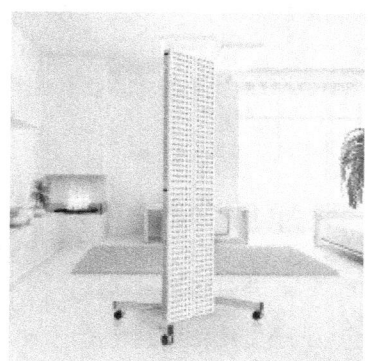

JOOVV Mobile Stand – Living Room

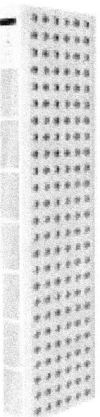

JOOVV SOLO – FRONT ANGLE

RESTORE

It's not a vitamin . . . it's not an herb . . . it's not a sleazy energy drink!

It's RESTORE!

Restore is a product conceived by a doctor by the name of Zach Bush. I love what this product has done for me so much that I feel Dr. Zach Bush is a personal friend.

I have been using Restore for a few years now, and the results are an iron-clad immune system and mental clarity, energy; you name it. Its function is to tighten the natural junction seams in your intestinal system to keep foreign toxic elements from entering the bloodstream and to be more easily eliminated from the body. As I and many others have said, we are continually assaulted by environmental toxins in the food, water, and air we take in on a daily basis.

We need stealth technology to guard against and defeat all this toxic crap being flung at us and Restore is it and the REAL DEAL!

This is basically fossilized dirt water with a twist of science. Don't get me wrong; it's a natural product.

It's not a prebiotic, and it's not a probiotic. It has "zoas" of untold proportions. And I mean protos . . . But a little goes a long way . . . drink it, nasal spray it, put in your ears . . . anywhere!

But enough! Go here - http://blog.restore4life.com
Be amazed and get well!

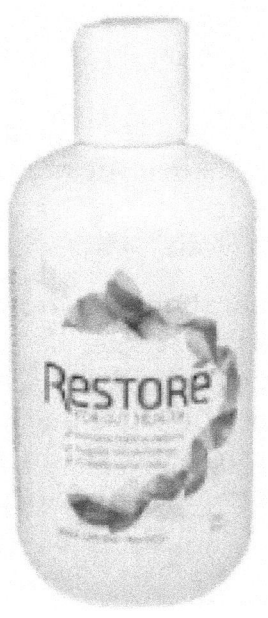

MOTHER DIRT

Mother dirt is a product designed to improve the bacterial environment on your skin that has been destroyed by the use of chemical soaps, creams, cosmetics, etcetera; as well as environmental toxins floating around in the air.

You can spray your whole body, but from my perspective, that could get a little expensive. Studies have shown, using *Mother Dirt* under your arms has reduced the need for deodorant. I really didn't try it much for that, but I did spray it on my face and other areas of my body. I found that my skin quality improved both in clarity and dryness without the use of cosmetic creams.

Give it a try! You will love it if you are seeking relief from the laurel sulfate cleansing world.

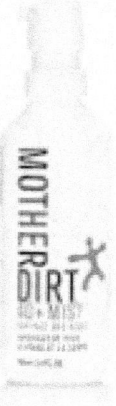

www.motherdirt.com

A SALTY SOLUTION

A Possible Asthma/COPD Killer!

This is truly an amazing thing, and I almost can't believe it myself, it's driving me crazy!

Not too long ago, a Salt Suite had opened in the nearby Mall around the corner from the house. I stopped by to investigate and spoke with the owner. He told me he was the first franchise outside of Florida and that the first therapy session was free . . . so I made an appointment and a week later checked it out. A large pink salt lamp lit the room and headphones were available with soothing music. Himalayan sea salt infused air came through the vents, and sitting there for roughly 40 minutes . . . just relaxed and breathed. I don't know if it was because I'm asthmatic, but the first 10 minutes I had problems breathing and then gradually relaxed and felt better for the duration. The after effects for me were good with generally better breathing, and I felt that my sinuses were more open. The owner had said that most of his clients, many of them children, had breathing issues, COPD etcetera.

The after effects for me were good with generally better breathing, and I felt that my sinuses were more open. On the contrary, my girlfriend felt like she had a sore throat and her nose hurt. The owner had said that most of his clients, many of them children, had breathing issues, COPD etcetera.

The store, being fairly new, was really busy. I don't know if it was because of the initial free sessions or all the repeat customers, but it's not really expensive - $99 for unlimited sessions for a month. Pretty reasonable. I was considering it, but it's difficult for me to get to anywhere at an appointed time with my busy schedule.

Still, it piqued my curiosity, and I checked into it online when I got home. I found a ceramic inhaler filled with pink Himalayan sea salt on Amazon and ordered it. It was only $15, and people were raving about it in the reviews; how it would help to relieve their asthma and COPD. They were astounded after a lifetime of asthma and breathing problems that they had stumbled upon something so simple and available forever. Why are doctors in the medical establishment not telling people about this?

Reading the history of the Himalayan salt mines, even the doctors back then use to take their patients into the caves to relieve their breathing problems! What!

I thought I had improved my asthmatic symptoms fairly remarkably up until I received this product and this just blew me away after using it for only several days and after a few weeks – wow! The progression of improvement was amazing!

I cannot recommend this product highly enough. The Himalayan pink salt inhaler by Natural Solutions is available at https://amzn.to/2IeQveX

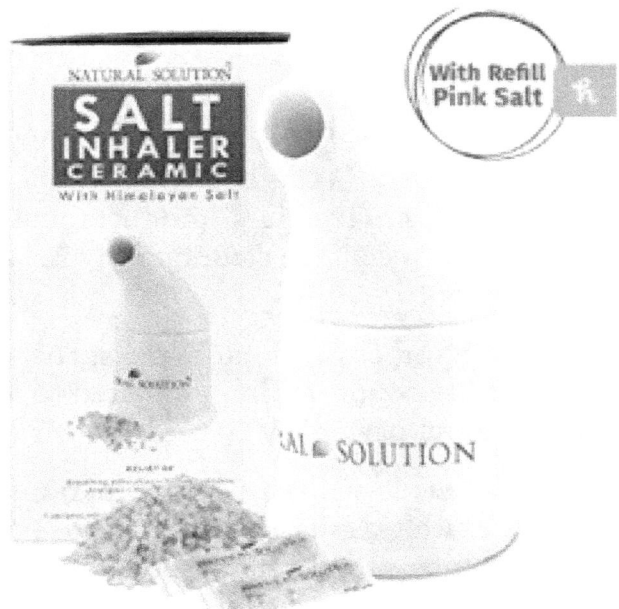

SUMMARY

In this book hopefully, you have found a pathway to unlock the secret to your own health. Here, in this book,
I have put forward the basic exercises, products and dietary methods that I have used to achieve a comparatively superior level of health at the age of 70.

If viewed as an anti-aging process, I would suppose that it would stand as the most credible counterpoint compared to any anti-aging tips and programs put forward by 20- and 30-year-olds.

So, this book is purely anecdotal in nature, summarizing my experiences over approximately the past 10 years. No peer reviews, and no bibliography except for some references to companies and products that I personally use.

Lastly, this is meant to be a primer or a handbook for you to pick and choose from whatever might work best for you and your circumstances. All exercises, nutritional
aspects, and movements are designed to be 5 to 10 minutes each and easily doable during the day with the exception of at least a 30-minute walk per day, to give you the energy to continue on and on.

FINAL NOTE

Although I do not represent or receive direct compensation from the companies or products mentioned in this book, there are some Amazon Associate links from which I would receive a small referral fee to hopefully cover the marketing costs of this book. The price is the same regardless. If that occurs, thank you in advance for your contribution.

Feel free to contact me at:

Gary@thecombinationofthings.com

with any comments, suggestions, or requests for further information or speaking engagements.

DISCLAIMER

All ideas, dietary suggestions, exercises and products are not intended to be replicated, used, practiced or pursued without first consulting your health care provider.

The author nor publisher are not liable or responsible for the consequences of acting upon any content in this book.

Any applications of the techniques, ideas, and suggestions in this book are at the reader's sole discretion and risk.